30-Day Meal Plan & Weight Loss Guide

ISBN: 9781796567410

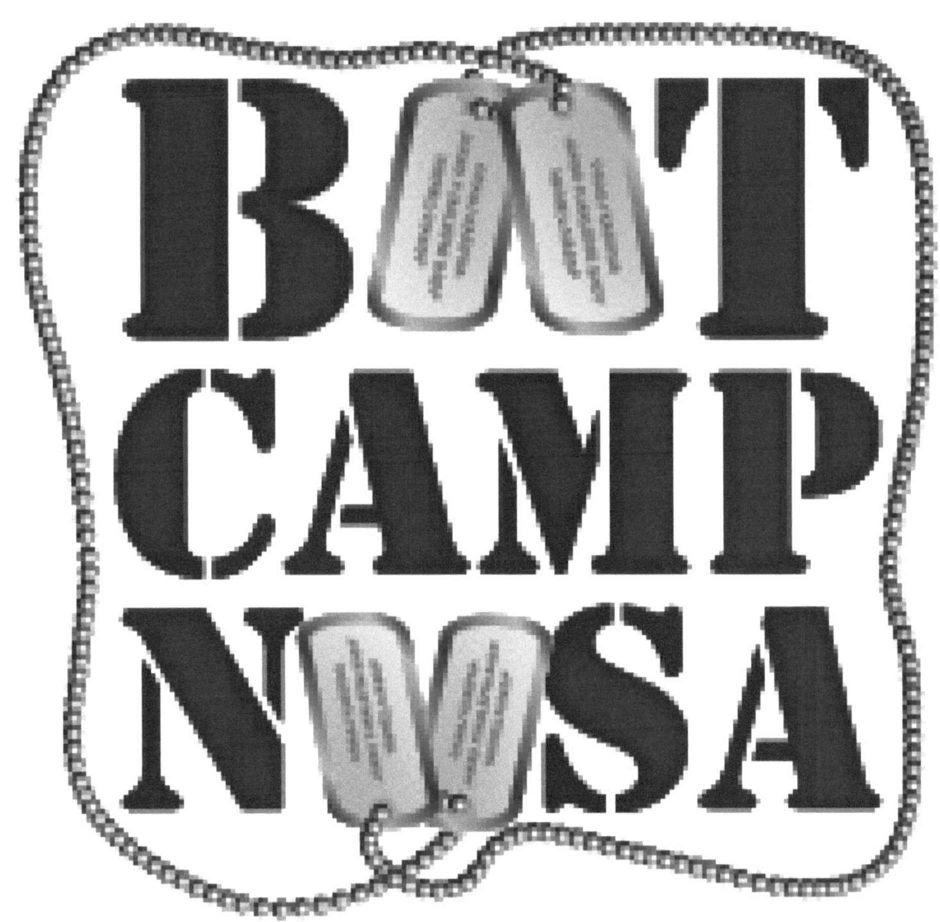

Presented by: Janjua Inc.

Bootcamp Noosa

30-Day Meal Plan & Weight Loss Guide

Table of Contents

Bootcamp Noosa
30-Day Meal Plan

A Successful Weight Loss Diet Starts from the Inside!

If you're like most people, you've been on a million weight loss diets, from Weight Watchers and Atkins to South Beach and celeb diets. You voraciously read magazines for their weight loss tips and gravitate toward the headlines that promise you can lose weight fast. The chances are good that you have, indeed, lost weight on many of these diets, but the chances are even better that you've gained it all back - plus some.

Weight Loss Diet Failure

You've probably bought into the propaganda that says you've failed at dieting; a different – and more accurate - way of looking at it is that the weight loss diet has failed you. That's because most diets focus on short-term changes that result in temporary weight loss, but never tackle the underlying factors that make you put on the pounds to begin with. In other words, they focus only on the "outside" problem - your body - and neglect everything below the surface - your emotions, your intellect, and your relationships. A diet for summer might work but you can bet by winter it will be back to haunt you again.

Turning Failure into Success

In order to lose weight and keep it off, you need a guide who will lead you on an exploratory journey to discover the power and control that you possess. Then, you need to be taught how to harness those powers to achieve all that you want in life - including fitting into your jeans again. You may have been told - either verbally or through insidious advertisements - that if you don't have power over your eating, you have no power at all. Nothing could be further from the truth. Every Person is magnificent, and every person has mental powers, emotional powers, social powers and physical powers just waiting to be tapped. When you heal your past wounds, and recognize and reinforce the power within you, you have laid the foundation for permanent weight loss.

Practical and Fun

If a weight loss diet is a drag, you'll never succeed in reaching your goals. On the other hand, if you have an empowering program to follow that is also practical and fun, you hold the keys to success. In fact, you can even drop a whole size in two weeks. The "secret" - if you want to call it that - is to adopt a well-tested exercise program that can instantly fit into your lifestyle. Remember, the success lies in simplicity, clarity, and practicality. Then, you need to adopt an eating plan that works synergistically with your exercise plan to build on the foundation of the inner work you have done in order to embrace your personal power. Remember that, with the right guide, you can do more than go on yet another weight loss diet; you can truly win in all areas of your life and achieve an outer beauty than matches your inner beauty.

Proven Weight Loss Tips

Australia has seen an enormous increase in the number of people considered obese by the medical community. In fact many call it an obesity epidemic. To combat this we find all sorts of pharmaceutical companies selling the "quick fix" pills, powders, and lotions that do nothing to actually help people take the fat off and keep it off.

Of course the same could be said of the diet industry as well. There are so many different diets going around now you could pick one a month and in a years time still have more to choose from.

What is truly needed are some sensible proven weight loss tips that people can implement no matter what their present physical condition is. That said let's dive right in.

#1 Drink more water. All too often Australians are borderline dehydrated and so their bodies are working on the water starvation reflex and not flushing the toxins and junk out.

#2 Eat more often. I bet you thought I was going to say eat less. While it is true that to lose weight you need to eat less calories than you expend...you need to eat more often to get the metabolic furnace stoked up and burning right. Get it out of starvation mode. So start the day off with breakfast. Even an instant breakfast drink and a piece of fruit as we head out the door in the morning.

#3 Move more. Depending on your physical condition you need to be moving more. Use the stairs rather than the elevator, park farther out from the office or the store, go for a walk around the block, go dancing, play with your kids. Make it fun. Running is not the only way to burn more calories.

#4 Finally, determine your "Why". Decide why you want to discard fat. Make your reason big enough to motivate you through the slumps that invariably happen.

Overcome Your Plateau with these 5 Easy Tips

If you need to lose a few extra pounds but feel you've hit a plateau, there are several ways to get your body back in the weight loss mode. A plateau is when you're no longer losing weight though it seems nothing has changed in your diet or exercise routine. Your body has adapted to the diet and now refuses to budge. So you must make some changes to boost your weight loss again.

These five free weight loss tips can help.

1. Change your calorie intake.

One way to overcome a plateau while maintaining a healthy weight loss plan is to change your calorie intake. Monitor how many calories you're eating and decrease them slightly to see if your weight scale moves again. You might try the zigzag method as well. To do this, decrease calories one day, and then increase calories the next. This helps shift your body out of its comfort zone. Only make minor adjustments and monitor your weight with each small change.

2. Replace a snack or two.

If you usually eat a chocolate bar as a mid-afternoon snack, try replacing this with a fruit or vegetable. Eat apples, bananas, carrots and low-fat dip, or celery and low-fat dip instead of chocolate. Fruits and vegetables are not only filling, but they also promote healthy weight loss.

3. Keep exercising, but endure longer.

Another way to boost weight loss and get your body moving again is to increase your exercise time. Instead of 30 minutes a day, try exercising 45 minutes a day. Walk every chance you get. Walking is a great (non-strenuous) exercise that helps your heart and promotes healthy weight loss. Park your car a little farther from the mall than usual when shopping. Walk your dog twice a day instead of only once. Take a walk during your breaks at work. These small changes can make a big difference in your weight loss efforts.

4. Monitor "what" you are eating.

Are you eating mainly sugar and carbohydrates on your weight loss diet? If so, try replacing one or two of these with a protein-rich food. Protein is a proven fat burner and energy booster, and many weight trainers use it to boost their workouts. Protein also helps you fill full longer so you're less likely to be hungry an hour later. There are protein snack bars on the market now so you can easily get a boost during the day. Other changes you can make include increasing your water and fiber intake if you feel you're not getting enough of these.

5. Eat smaller, more frequent meals.

Instead of eating three large meals a day, try eating smaller, more frequent meals. Reduce portion sizes at your regular meals, and add small snacks in between each meal. This helps boost your metabolism and keeps you from being hungry during the day and splurging at night. Keep in mind that fast weight loss can be unhealthy, but you might lose fast at the start of any diet or when overcoming a plateau. This is normal. These tips are to help you break the plateau so you can start losing weight again. Weight loss diets can help you feel and look better than you ever have before. Use these ideas to break through your plateau today so you can reach your future weight loss goals.

How to Choose a Weight Loss Plan

Whether you need to lose only a few extra Kg's or up to 20 or 60kg's, you can become weary while trying to choose among the hundreds of weight loss plans available. There are plenty of weight loss diets that involve eating special foods, drinking certain drink mixtures, or taking weight loss pills. But which one's right for you? Use these tips to choose the weight loss diet that will fit your lifestyle and daily routine.

What's Your Style?

A weight loss diet plan should fit your style. What works for one person may or may not work for you. You must consider your daily routine, the types of foods you like, and what your body needs. Do you enjoy sweets? Do you enjoy eating meats? There are a number of diets that allow you to eat meats and sweets in moderation. Also, consider how many meals you can eat. Do you normally eat three square meals per day, or do you take smaller, more frequent meals? These are questions to ask before starting a weight loss plan so you can find a diet that's easy to stay with to reach your goals.

Study the Risks

Some diets are more risky than others when it comes to weight loss and your health. For instance, fast weight loss can be harmful to the body, especially if continued over a long period of time. Weight loss pills can be dangerous too if taken without first consulting a physician. Some diets are harmful to the body if you have certain health conditions. For instance, a diet that emphasizes meat might not be best if you already have digestive problems or heart problems. If you have any serious health problems or are taking prescription medications, you should talk with your doctor before starting a weight loss diet.

Types of Weight Loss Diets

There are many weight loss plans, but each is different. It's a good idea to study the different types of plans before getting started on your weight loss journey. Find the type of weight loss diet that best suits you. Consider how each affects your body and health, and how each plan fits into your schedule or routine. Let's see what types of diet plans are available and what is required with each.

Diets for Fast Weight Loss

Though fast weight loss is not recommended for the long term, there are some quick diets to help you lose 2-6kgs in no time. These include the low-carb diet, three-to-five-day meal replacement shakes, water or juice fasts, and alternate vegetable/fruit diets in which you eat only fruits one day and only vegetables the next. These diets work great for a quick fix, but are very difficult (and possibly unhealthy) to maintain for the long term.

Low Calorie Weight Loss Diets

There are many low calorie diets with which you will reduce your daily calories to lose weight. There are several ways to monitor your calories. You can read food labels and count the calories of everything you eat. You can also use a calorie guide to determine how many calories are in certain foods or dishes that do not have labels. Weight Watchers provides an easy point counter that calculates points based on calories, fiber, and fat grams in foods.

Fixed Menu Plans

With a fixed menu diet plan, you will be given a list of all the foods you can eat. The meal plans are put together especially for you based on your likes and needs. This type of diet can make things easy for you as you lose weight, but keep in mind that you will eventually need to start planning your own meals again. So it's a good idea to learn how to plan your meals after you've lost the initial weight. This will help you keep the weight off once the fixed-menu diet has ended.

Exchange Food Diet

With an exchange food diet, you will plan meals with a set number of servings from several food groups. The foods are determined by calorie intake, and you can pick and choose among foods that have the same calories to give you a variety of choices at each meal. This diet is great if you've just completed a fixed menu diet because it allows you to make your own food choices each day.

Low Fat Diet

Another type of diet is the low fat diet, which requires lowering the intake of fat. This doesn't mean eating fat-free everything, but simply lowering fats (especially saturated fats) and oils to a normal level according to the food pyramid. Fat should take up around 30 percent of the calories eaten. Lowering saturated fat promotes healthy weight loss and helps lower cholesterol levels to promote good heart

health. There are many foods that advertise "low fat" but many of these are also very high in sugar. Look for foods that are low in fat and low in sugar for healthy weight loss. Also, limit fast foods or make healthier choices from the menu such as salads or grilled foods. Many fried fast foods are loaded with fat.

Weight Loss through Reduced Portions

There are also weight loss diets with which only the portions are reduced, but you basically eat anything you want. You eat only small portions of foods and basically follow your stomach. When your stomach is empty, you eat slowly until you feel satisfied, but not overly full. You only eat when you're really hungry. This type of diet gives you freedom to choose what you want to eat, but limits how much you can eat. The concept is when you eat less food in smaller portions then you're also eating less fat and calories with every meal, no matter what the food.

There are also pre-packaged meals and formulas to help promote weight loss. Almost any diet can work if you adhere to its rules, add activity or exercises, and drink plenty of water. Study each type of diet to find one that will work for you, and check with you doctor before starting a new diet plan if you have a health condition or take medications. You can easily research diet plans online and find many free weight loss tips to help you develop a plan.

Boost Metabolism And Lose Weight By Eating Well

We've all known for some time that breakfast is an integral part of the day. Now research has shown that, regardless of physical activity, eating high fibre cereal in the morning at least three times a week leads to having a lower body mass index. This study followed 2,300 teenage girls over ten years, and was conducted by the National Heart, Lung and Blood Institute in the US. One reason people skip breakfast is because they are trying to reduce their overall calorie intake. Whilst its important not to eat too many excess calories, having breakfast, even if its a simple smoothie, or a couple of pieces of fruit, will reduce the urge to snack on chocolate or other unhealthy options, as well as improving your performance at work and reducing fatigue. Sometimes its not just the overall calorie intake, but the types of foods we eat as well. Grab a couple of carrots instead of some toast - not only will you be getting fiber, but the phytochemicals such as carotene and other vitamins will help you get the most out of your body and your day. And if you're a bit disorganized with buying fruit and vegetables, visit the local fruit street vendor on the way to your local coffee shop before work. It beats a muffin nutritionally.

And for the final word on going overboard with calorie restriction, recent research found that even though mice will live up to 50% longer by eating less, humans don't. The most having a low calorie diet over your life would do is extend your time span on this earth by 7% Physiologically, having breakfast will in fact boost your metabolism. And its certainly a cheaper way to do that than investing in a bottle of diet pills.

A couple of weight loss tips for parents and expecting mothers.

Early research has suggested that those mothers who eat excessively (think Britney Spears) have children who are more prone to being overweight by the time they are toddlers. This sets up food difficulties from a young age. And beware of teenagers or children who develop poor eating habits, combined with sedentary activities like playing playstation or xbox games too much, and watching television at the expense of even non-athletic activities like having a job or joining school clubs. These kids will have a greater tendency of growing into overweight or obese adults. One key to integrating changes in your diet, whether with the goal of losing weight, or simply being more healthy, is to add variety. Its easy to get into a food rut, stuck for something tasty to eat that is also going to support our goals.

Planning ahead, and doing a little research, can be one way of mitigating those moments when the urge to grab something unhealthy is driven by both hunger and unappetizing dishes. Eating fruit and vegetables raw gives you many of their vitamins undiminished by cooking processes. It also means you get enzymes which are great for helping the digestive process. Watermelon is rich in vitamin C and is also one of the few sources of lycopene, others being tomatoes, red grapefruit and guava. Lycopene is a particularly effective antioxidant.

Lose Weight Tricks

Thousands of people are looking for lose weight tricks which can help them with their ongoing struggle. All over the world people are looking for some answers which can make the difference between a frustrating struggle to lose weight, and smooth steady progress. Here are some lose weight tricks designed to help you find the right path.

Lose Weight Tricks 1

If you are determined to lose weight, you have got to stick at it. Nothing great was ever achieved without some effort, and possibly the odd sacrifice. Don't worry if you think it is all taking too long. Time seems to go very quickly in our busy world, so before you know it you will be where you want to be. The time will pass anyway, so make use of it to create a better and healthier you.

Lose Weight Tricks 2

Reward yourself when you achieve major targets. It is a time tested psychological trick to give yourself small treats as a reward when you achieve something significant. Losing your first five Kgs is a vital landmark, for example, so go and visit your favorite restaurant to celebrate. Of course you need to exercise some restraint when you get there, but you are more likely to do this when you are full of satisfaction having reached a significant target!

Lose Weight Tricks 3

Eat a lot of salad food. There are virtually no calories in salad, but plenty of water and nutrients. Salad will allow you to still eat decent sized meals and not feel hungry, but reduce the number of empty calories you take in. This can be extremely beneficial, as most people's calorie intake is too high.

Lose Weight Tricks 4

If you have sugar in tea or coffee, try to cut down on the number of cups you drink. Many people find themselves routinely drinking five or six cups of coffee or tea a day, and if these have sugar in, you are taking in and extra couple of hundred calories you don't need. You can take these two hundred calories in a healthier form, or cut them out altogether to help you lose weight.

Weight Loss: Setting Reasonable Long Term Goals

We see a lot of people struggling with weight issues and their body image. With the available resources and materials for weight loss spilled all over the place, those, who are overweight, are a bit confused about which method to follow to shed those extra lbs. Although the basics of weight loss do not change, they depend on setting realistic goals, cutting the calorie intake and exercising a little bit. Many presume that a weight loss program is all about a restricted diet, or fad diets, or diet pills and involving strenuous physical exercises. But, actually the basics of weight loss program are rational, flexible and healthy to which any one can adhere to while they work well on the person aiming to lose weight.

The first basic step towards weight loss is to set a reachable goal. When setting a goal to reduce weight, it is good to know the reason for doing so, benefits you may get at the end of the weight reduction program and the changes you are willing to make in your diet. This kind of analysis of the self helps understand the problem the better way and helps in setting realistic goals for weight loss. The weight loss efforts should be a reasonable one and should be gradual. Once the goal is set to reduce say 1kg a week, then comes the step of creating a food journal to analyze and monitor what you eat for the particular week. This food journal helps keep track of what you eat, or drink. Sometimes the feeling towards the food you eat is also jotted down. This is very important as it throws light on the food pattern and habits of the person. The weight loss is also recorded. By reviewing the food pattern, the foods that needed to be avoided can be seen clearly and can be substituted with healthy foods.

The secret is to be very consistent with this surely you will see positive results. Water is a very good natural hunger suppressant and can be taken in good quantities, if you note that you are drinking less amounts of water. It too can contribute to the weight loss efforts.

When the diet is combined with good exercise say walking or swimming or aerobics, it too aids in burning calories. The exercise should be in such a way that when it is done, it should be enjoyable, choose the kind of activity which interests you a lot than slogging. Exercise too needs to be tracked in the journal to see its effects with your own eyes.

30-Day Meal Plan

<u>Daily Meal Plan 1</u>

Meal 1 (Breakfast) A Whole Egg with oatmeal and Small Glass of Skim Milk

Snack 1 (Mid-Morning) Low Sugar Strawberry Yogurt used for dipping Banana

Meal 2 (Lunch) Turkey Breast with Brown Rice

Snack 2 (Late Afternoon) Low Sugar Strawberry Yogurt used for dipping Banana

Meal 3 (Dinner) Grilled Tuna with Asparagus

Snack 3 (Late Evening) Small Handful of Unsalted Walnuts on Small Salad

<u>Daily Meal Plan 2</u>

Meal 1 (Breakfast) Cream of Wheat with Glass of Skim Milk

Snack 1 (Mid-Morning) Low-Fat Cottage Cheese with Blueberries

Meal 2 (Lunch) Whole Wheat wrap with Turkey and Low-Fat Cheese

Snack 2 (Late Afternoon) Low-Fat Cottage Cheese with Blueberries

Meal 3 (Dinner) Baked Chicken Breast with Broccoli

Snack 3 (Late Evening) A Low-Fat Cheese Stick with a Few Celery Sticks

<u>Daily Meal Plan 3</u>

Meal 1 (Breakfast) Oatmeal with Skim Milk

Snack 1 (Mid-Morning) ½ Banana with Low-Fat Yogurt

Meal 2 (Lunch) Grilled Chicken Breast with small sweet potato

Snack 2 (Late Afternoon) Apple with ¼ handful of unsalted almonds

Meal 3 (Dinner) Grilled Salmon with Asparagus

Snack 3 (Late Evening) Celery Sticks

Daily Meal Plan 4

Meal 1 (Breakfast) Turkey Bacon with Egg and Whole Grain Toast

Snack 1 (Mid-Morning) Can of Tuna with Watermelon

Meal 2 (Lunch) Grilled Chicken on Bed of Salad Greens with Whole Grain Crackers

Snack 2 (Late Afternoon) Mango with Low-Fat Cheese Sticks

Meal 3 (Dinner) Broiled Salmon with Green Salad

Snack 3 (Late Evening) Celery Sticks w/ small Amount of Natural Peanut Butter

Daily Meal Plan 5

Meal 1 (Breakfast) 2 Slices of Whole Grain Bread, a Whole Egg and some Egg Whites

Snack 1 (Mid-Morning) Peaches with Low-Sugar Yogurt

Meal 2 (Lunch) Sweet Potato with Broiled Turkey Burgers

Snack 2 (Late Afternoon) Can of Tuna with Watermelon

Meal 3 (Dinner) Baked Tilapia with Cold Spinach Salad

Snack 3 (Late Evening) Plain Low Fat Yogurt used as Dip for Veggie Sticks

Daily Meal Plan 6

Meal 1 (Breakfast) Slice of whole grain bread w/ teaspoon of peanut butter and Medium Glass of Low Fat or Skim Milk

Snack 1 (Mid-Morning) Mango with Low-Fat Cheese Sticks

Meal 2 (Lunch) Whole Wheat Pasta with Boiled Shrimp

Snack 2 (Late Afternoon) Bit of High Fiber Whole Grain Cereal mixed w/low sugar apple sauce + Walnuts

Meal 3 (Dinner) Grilled Chicken Breast with Sliced Cucumbers

Snack 3 (Late Evening) Plain Low Fat Yogurt used as Dip for Veggie Sticks

Daily Meal Plan 7

Meal 1 (Breakfast) Healthy higher fiber cold cereal with low fat or Skim milk

Snack 1 (Mid-Morning) A Couple of Low Fat Cheese Sticks and a Mango

Meal 2 (Lunch) Grilled Tilapia with a Small Serving of Whole Wheat Pasta

Snack 2 (Late Afternoon) 1 Cup of Low Sugar Yogurt with Strawberries

Meal 3 (Dinner) Grilled Turkey Breast with Cooked Spinach with Dash of Vinegar

Snack 3 (Late Evening) Small serving of Canned Chicken with a Sliced Cucumber

Daily Meal Plan 8

Meal 1 (Breakfast) Plain Oatmeal with a whole egg and some egg whites

Snack 1 (Mid-Morning) Half a handful of unsalted almonds and a half handful of blueberries

Meal 2 (Lunch) Grilled Tuna Steak with a Medium Sweet Potato

Snack 2 (Late Afternoon) Low Fat Cottage Cheese with pineapple

Meal 3 (Dinner) Chicken and Shrimp Stir Fry with Vegetable Medley

Snack 3 (Late Evening) A Small Can of Tuna with some Raw Veggies

Daily Meal Plan 9

Meal 1 (Breakfast) Whole Wheat Wrap with Peanut Butter and Small Glass of Skim Milk

Snack 1 (Mid-Morning) Half a handful of unsalted almonds and small apple

Meal 2 (Lunch) 1 Peanut Butter sandwich on whole grain bread

Snack 2 (Late Afternoon) 1 cup of lower sugar yogurt with a peach

Meal 3 (Dinner) Grilled Turkey Burgers with Grilled Veggie Kabobs

Snack 3 (Late Evening) A Low Fat Cheese Stick with some Cucumber Slices

Daily Meal Plan 10

Meal 1 (Breakfast) Healthy higher fiber cold cereal with low fat or Skim milk

Snack 1 (Mid-Morning) 1 cup of lower sugar yogurt with a banana

Meal 2 (Lunch) 1 turkey sandwich (lots of turkey) with low fat cheese on whole grain bread

Snack 2 (Late Afternoon) Half a handful of unsalted almonds and small pear

Meal 3 (Dinner) Grilled Turkey Burgers with Grilled Veggie Kabobs

Snack 3 (Late Evening) Celery Sticks with a small spread of Peanut Butter

Daily Meal Plan 11

Meal 1 (Breakfast) 1 Whole Egg, ½ Chicken Breast, and 1 Slice of Whole Grain Bread

Snack 1 (Mid-Morning) Unsalted Almonds with Pear

Meal 2 (Lunch) 1 chicken breast sandwich on whole wheat/grain w/mustard and w/out mayo

Snack 2 (Late Afternoon) Apple Slices with teaspoon Peanut Butter

Meal 3 (Dinner) Grilled Halibut with Cooked Zucchini and Yellow Squash

Snack 3 (Late Evening) Celery Sticks with Plain low-sugar yogurt for dipping

Daily Meal Plan 12

Meal 1 (Breakfast) Cream of Wheat with 1 Whole Egg

Snack 1 (Mid-Morning) Walnuts (Unsalted) with an Orange

Meal 2 (Lunch) Mozzarella and tomato sandwich (Whole wheat or grain)

Snack 2 (Late Afternoon) Half a handful of Unsalted Pecans and a half handful of Cherries

Meal 3 (Dinner) Lean grilled pork chops w/ green beans

Snack 3 (Late Evening) Cucumber Sticks w/plain Yogurt for Dipping

Daily Meal Plan 13

Meal 1 (Breakfast) Oatmeal with Turkey Bacon small glass of Skim Milk

Snack 1 (Mid-Morning) ½ Handful Unsalted Almonds with Pear

Meal 2 (Lunch) Peanut butter and banana sandwich on whole wheat or grain bread

Snack 2 (Late Afternoon) Half a handful of unsalted Pecans and an Orange

Meal 3 (Dinner) Grilled chicken breast and asparagus

Snack 3 (Late Evening) Raw Cauliflower Sticks w/teaspoon of low fat Dip

Daily Meal Plan 14

Meal 1 (Breakfast) Healthy higher fiber cold cereal with low fat or Skim milk

Snack 1 (Mid-Morning) A Couple of Low Fat Cheese Sticks and a large Orange

Meal 2 (Lunch) 1 Tablespoon Almond Butter on whole grain or wheat crackers

Snack 2 (Late Afternoon) Low Fat Cottage Cheese with a small Papaya

Meal 3 (Dinner) Unsalted Pecans on Green Salad with Oil and Vinegar Dressing

Snack 3 (Late Evening) Raw Broccoli Sticks w/teaspoon of low fat Dip

Daily Meal Plan 15

Meal 1 (Breakfast) A Whole Grain English Muffin w/slice of low-fat cheese and Small Glass of Skim Milk

Snack 1 (Mid-Morning) A Peach and a large teaspoon scoop of Peanut Butter

Meal 2 (Lunch) Black Beans and Rice (brown or wild rice)

Snack 2 (Late Afternoon) Low Sugar Plain Yogurt used for dipping Peach Slices

Meal 3 (Dinner) Grilled Shrimp with Asparagus and Mushrooms

Snack 3 (Late Evening) Small Handful of Unsalted Pecans on Small Salad

Daily Meal Plan 16

Meal 1 (Breakfast) A Whole Grain English Muffin w/peanut butter spread and Small Glass of Skim Milk

Snack 1 (Mid-Morning) Apple Slices with Almond Butter spread

Meal 2 (Lunch) Red Beans and Rice (brown or wild rice)

Snack 2 (Late Afternoon) Low Sugar Plain Yogurt used for dipping Apple Slices

Meal 3 (Dinner) Baked Scallops with Cabbage

Snack 3 (Late Evening) Small Handful of Unsalted Walnuts on Small Salad

Daily Meal Plan 17

Meal 1 (Breakfast) A Bran Cereal w/Skim Milk

Snack 1 (Mid-Morning) Pineapple with Low Fat Cottage Cheese

Meal 2 (Lunch) Pinto Beans and 2 Slices Whole Grain Toast

Snack 2 (Late Afternoon) Low Sugar Blueberry Yogurt and a Plum

Meal 3 (Dinner) Grilled Grouper with Fresh Onion, Cucumber, and Tomato Slices

Snack 3 (Late Evening) Small Low Sugar Yogurt and Celery Sticks

Daily Meal Plan 18

Meal 1 (Breakfast) Puffed Wheat Cereal w/Skim Milk

Snack 1 (Mid-Morning) Mandarin Orange w/large teaspoon scoop of Almond Butter

Meal 2 (Lunch) No Skin Cornish Hen with Sweet Potato

Snack 2 (Late Afternoon) Nectarine w/ strawberry yogurt

Meal 3 (Dinner) Small Filet Mignon w/Mushrooms and Cold Spinach Salad

Snack 3 (Late Evening) Fresh Carrot Sticks w/Plain Yogurt Dip

Daily Meal Plan 19

Meal 1 (Breakfast) Shredded Wheat Cereal w/Skim Milk

Snack 1 (Mid-Morning) Nectarine w/large teaspoon scoop of Peanut Butter

Meal 2 (Lunch) No Skin, White Meat Rotisserie Chicken w/Brown Rice

Snack 2 (Late Afternoon) Mandarin Orange w/ blueberry yogurt

Meal 3 (Dinner) Lean Flank Steak w/Cooked Summer Squash and Zucchini

Snack 3 (Late Evening) Fresh Broccoli Sticks with Plain Yogurt Dip

Daily Meal Plan 20

Meal 1 (Breakfast) Whole Grain Waffles with Turkey Bacon and a Glass of Skim Milk

Snack 1 (Mid-Morning) Handful of Blackberries and Vanilla Yogurt

Meal 2 (Lunch) Green Salad w/Egg Whites, Cucumbers, & Tomatoes & Whole Wheat

Crackers plus Olive Oil and Vinegar Based Dressing

Snack 2 (Late Afternoon) A Pear and a Handful of Almonds

Meal 3 (Dinner) Turkey Sausage (low sodium) with Sauerkraut

Snack 3 (Late Evening) Cucumber Slices w/hot sauce and a few Unsalted Walnuts

Daily Meal Plan 21

Meal 1 (Breakfast) High Fiber Cereal with Skim Milk

Snack 1 (Mid-Morning) Handful of Blueberries and Plain Yogurt

Meal 2 (Lunch) Green Salad w/Almonds, Cucumbers, & Tomatoes & Whole Wheat
Crackers

plus Olive Oil and Vinegar Based Dressing

Snack 2 (Late Afternoon) Low Fat Yogurt and Papaya

Meal 3 (Dinner) Chicken Sausage (low sodium) with Sauerkraut

Snack 3 (Late Evening) Cucumber Slices w/a few Unsalted Almonds

Daily Meal Plan 22

Meal 1 (Breakfast) 1 Egg Yolk and 2 Egg Whites w Whole Grain Toast

Snack 1 (Mid-Morning) Handful of Strawberries and Vanilla Yogurt

Meal 2 (Lunch) Green Salad w/Pecans, Cucumbers, & Tomatoes & Whole Wheat Crackers plus Olive Oil and Vinegar Based Dressing

Snack 2 (Late Afternoon) 2 Plums with a Small Handful of Pecans

Meal 3 (Dinner) Kidney Beans w/Grilled Eggplant and Fresh Tomato Slices

Snack 3 (Late Evening) Cucumber Slices w/a few Unsalted Pecans

Daily Meal Plan 23

Meal 1 (Breakfast) Kashi Cereal with Low Fat or Skim Milk

Snack 1 (Mid-Morning) Handful of Cherries and Plain Yogurt

Meal 2 (Lunch) Grilled Chicken Breast on a Green Salad w/Oil & Vinegar Dressing

Snack 2 (Late Afternoon) Apple w/Peanut Butter

Meal 3 (Dinner) Eggs and Fresh Salsa with Sliced Cucumbers

Snack 3 (Late Evening) Veggie Sticks and Low Fat Yogurt

Daily Meal Plan 24

Meal 1 (Breakfast) Turkey Bacon, Whole Grain Toast and a Glass of Skim Milk

Snack 1 (Mid-Morning) Handful of Unsalted Almonds and 1/2 Handful of Fresh Strawberries

Meal 2 (Lunch) Grilled Turkey Burgers w/Brown Rice

Snack 2 (Late Afternoon) Mango Slices and ½ handful of Peanuts

Meal 3 (Dinner) Homemade Chicken and Vegetable Soup

Snack 3 (Late Evening) Cucumber Slices w/ hot sauce w/small handful or Pecans

Daily Meal Plan 25

Meal 1 (Breakfast) Whole Egg w/ Egg Whites and a Whole Grain Waffle

Snack 1 (Mid-Morning) Low Fat Cottage Cheese with Peaches

Meal 2 (Lunch) Chicken Fajitas w/Corn or Whole Wheat Tortillas w/ Wild Rice

Snack 2 (Late Afternoon) ½ Handful of Walnuts w/an Orange

Meal 3 (Dinner) Homemade Turkey and Vegetable Soup

Snack 3 (Late Evening) Low Fat Yogurt used for Dipping Veggie Sticks

Daily Meal Plan 26

Meal 1 (Breakfast) Plain Oatmeal and one Slice of Whole Grain Toast w/teaspoon of peanut butter

Snack 1 (Mid-Morning) Low Fat Cheese Stick and Papaya

Meal 2 (Lunch) Grilled Fish with Sweet Potato

Snack 2 (Late Afternoon) 1 Cup of Low Sugar Yogurt with Kiwi

Meal 3 (Dinner) Baked Chicken with Steamed Asparagus

Snack 3 (Late Evening) Small Green Salad w/Small handful of Walnuts

Daily Meal Plan 27

Meal 1 (Breakfast) Cream of Wheat, Multi Grain Toast and Small Glass of Skim Milk

Snack 1 (Mid-Morning) ½ Handful of Peanuts and Mandarin Oranges

Meal 2 (Lunch) Whole Wheat Turkey Wrap w/Oil & Vinegar Based Dressing

Snack 2 (Late Afternoon) Watermelon

Meal 3 (Dinner) Green Salad w/Grilled Chicken Breast and Oil & Vinegar Dressing

Snack 3 (Late Evening) 1 Cup of Low Fat Blueberry Yogurt w/small green salad

Daily Meal Plan 28

Meal 1 (Breakfast) Whole Grain English Muffin w/Low Fat Cheese and Small Glass of Skim Milk

Snack 1 (Mid-Morning) Low Fat Cottage Cheese w/Blueberries

Meal 2 (Lunch) Peanut Butter Sandwich on Whole Grain Bread

Snack 2 (Late Afternoon) Banana Slices w/Peanut Butter

Meal 3 (Dinner) Lean Grilled Pork Chops with Grilled Squash and Zucchini

Snack 3 (Late Evening) Cucumber Slices w/Low Fat Yogurt Used for Dipping

Daily Meal Plan 29

Meal 1 (Breakfast) Unsweetened Natural Granola w/Skim Milk

Snack 1 (Mid-Morning) Strawberries and ½ Handful of Almonds

Meal 2 (Lunch) Kashi Bar with Yogurt

Snack 2 (Late Afternoon) Pear Slices with Peanut Butter spread

Meal 3 (Dinner) Spinach Salad w/Oil & Vinegar Based Dressing w/ Broiled Turkey Burgers

Snack 3 (Late Evening) 1 Cup of Low Fat Plain Yogurt w/cold raw carrots

Daily Meal Plan 30

Meal 1 (Breakfast) Cream of Wheat and Turkey Bacon

Snack 1 (Mid-Morning) Papaya and 1 Low Fat Cheese Stick

Meal 2 (Lunch) Chicken Fajitas and Small Green Salad with corn or whole wheat tortillas

Snack 2 (Late Afternoon) Grapes & ½ Handful of Walnuts

Meal 3 (Dinner) Grilled Salmon w/Steamed Vegetable Medley

Snack 3 (Late Evening) Veggie Sticks w/Low Fat Yogurt

Obesity is epidemic in the United States. The number of overweight and obese Americans has grown at a disturbing rate, especially over the past few years, to the point where today more Americans are overweight than are normal weight. In fact, over sixty percent of Americans are now considered to be overweight, with over 30 percent of the population considered to be obese (e.g., overweight by more than 20-30% of recommended weight). These numbers describe a tragic public health situation. Being overweight increases a person's risk of serious illness. A very large (and growing) percentage of citizens are at increased risk for developing serious chronic diseases, and face the prospect of early disability or death as the result of being overweight. Meanwhile the entire society struggles under the burden of the resulting increase in health care costs.

Obesity

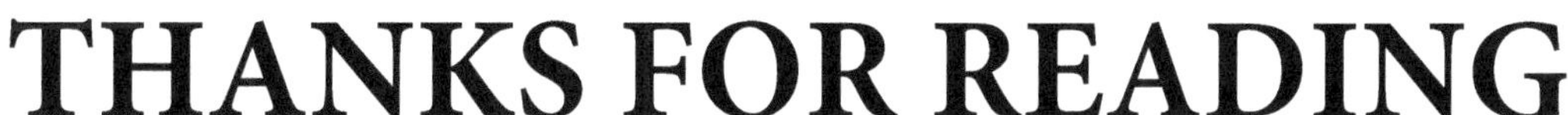

THANKS FOR READING

Muhammad Naeem Janjua

Shazaimbooki@yahoo.com

www.ingramcontent.com/pod-product-compliance
Lightning Source LLC
Chambersburg PA
CBHW041136260726
48664CB00027B/1264